T0147006

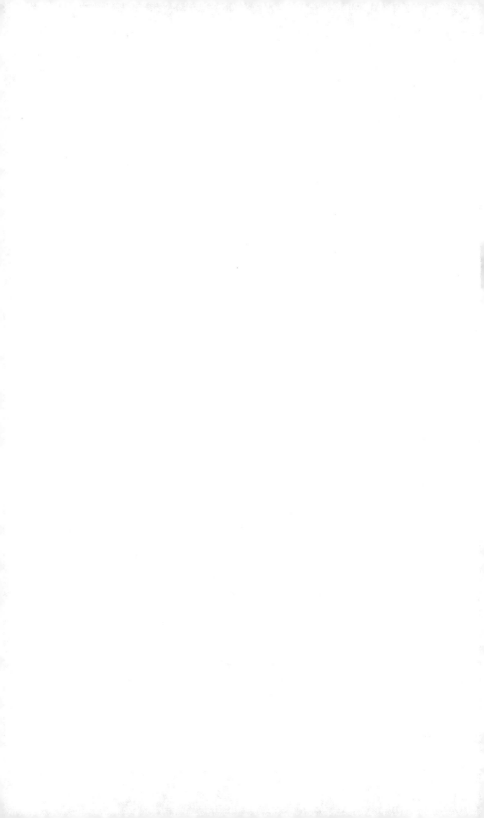

MASTERING

Beauty

STEPHANIA PARENT PH.D.

BALBOA.
PRESS
A DIVISION OF HAY HOUSE

Interior Graphics/Art Credit: Stephania Parent

Balboa Press books may be ordered through booksellers or by contacting:

Balboa Press
A Division of Hay House
1663 Liberty Drive
Bloomington, IN 47403
www.balboapress.com
1 (877) 407-4847

Print information available on the last page.

ISBN: 978-1-9822-1368-8 (sc)
ISBN: 978-1-9822-1369-5 (e)

Balboa Press rev. date: 10/19/2018

For my daughter Laila Avalon

Your strength, determination, confidence, and
majestic light inspire me every day.
Always let your light shine bright.

I love you!

CONTENTS

Special thanks to:

My editor Mischa Geracoulis for her patience, talent, encouragement and support.

PREFACE

Beauty in its purest form may perhaps best be seen and appreciated in that of a newborn baby. A baby that has come straight from Heaven into the arms of its new mother is a beautiful thing. Babies represent the purity, beauty, love, joy, innocence, potential, and grace in us all. It has been said that the sweet smell of a newborn baby is that of Heaven because their souls are still very closely connected to God.

As we grow older we all strive to hold onto our youthful appearance and beauty, as we tend to associate our external looks with who we are. We attach ourselves to this look and that cream as a way of trying to look good. We think that if we look good our experiences in life will improve. This is partially true, but it isn't a strategy that will work for anyone in the long run without a strong spiritual foundation. Because as we all know life is filled with pits and valleys, and when we are in the pits it doesn't matter how much retail therapy you give yourself or what new makeup you buy, it will not help you feel better on the inside.

Those values that newborn babies represent are in us all! But over time we have forgotten our true beauty, the beauty that we are all born with. The love, potential, grace, and everlasting joy are there looking right back at you; it just needs to be called back, or forth, if you will.

I have been working in the beauty industry for over twenty years, and I love beauty in all its splendor. My standards are probably considered high, as I really love to put my face on, fix my hair, and wear a nice outfit! There's nothing wrong with taking time to respect ourselves and try and look our best, but I have found that whenever I have been in the pits, which seemed pretty often working as a freelance artist, it wasn't my makeup tips and tricks that pulled me out and up to the valley—although looking my best helped a little! What helped was my consistent and thoughtful prayer and meditation practice.

So that is what this book is about! Mastering Beauty is a daily workbook that will give you insight, tips, and techniques to help you look and feel your best every day, and help you to recreate your own true beauty and successful life through the power of mindful meditation.

CHAPTER 1

Beginning Your Journey

You are beautiful! Sit in a comfortable seated position either in a chair or even better on a meditation cushion with your legs crossed underneath you, with your spine elongated and straight. Allow your hands to rest folded onto your lap gently, then close your eyes and simply imagine now a beautiful bright light pulsating out from the center of your chest where your heart is. Begin to breathe in and out slowly.

Focus on your breath, feel it moving in and out. Then as you relax, begin to imagine that beautiful light growing bigger and brighter, surrounding your body. Let the light continue to expand until it fills, then surrounds, the room you are in. With your breath push the light out into the unknown, the space between Heaven and Earth, and exhale gently. Rest here, and be still now. Congratulations! You have just taken the first step towards complete and ultimate beauty! Because it starts from the inside with the power of meditation.

CHAPTER 2

Beauty Sleep

Last night I woke up in the middle of the night, which I have frequently done throughout my life. Once upon a time when I was up and couldn't get back to sleep, I would spend a few hours worrying about this job or that guy, trying to put my life in order while mentally doing a workout session. Eventually I would fall back asleep, but would always wake up the next morning feeling as if I had gained 10 pounds between my ears! Sound familiar?

Up at night and can't sleep? Did you know that when we are in a deep sleep our souls often leave our bodies to refresh and rejuvenate much like our bodies and minds do while we are asleep? Without regular, healthy sleep we cannot fully be present to live at our fullest potential. Among all of the numerous health benefits that a good night's sleep provides, it also puts us in a subconscious state of spiritual receptivity in which we can more easily receive guidance and communication from our dreams, spirit guides, and loved ones.

Having a dream journal beside your bedside table is a great way to remember your dreams and messages from spirit. You can experiment by being specific in asking your spirit guides and loved ones by writing down a question on a piece of paper and putting it under your pillow. See what happens in your dreams. Often, the very next day a solution will be presented to you. This is a technique that I've successfully used to help me switch off the mental exercises and get back to sleep.

As you are lying down, focus your breath in the middle of your chest where your heart is, and feel your chest move up and down. Continue to breathe, and if your mind starts to race again, immediately shift your attention back to your breathing. You can begin counting slowly as you breathe, on 1 inhale on 2 exhale etcetera. This exercise is called a sleep meditation and it will help you fall asleep and stay asleep as you welcome in the source of your being. Be patient and give yourself time to get use to these new techniques. If you are consistent, you will soon be enjoying the beauty of a good night's sleep.

CHAPTER 3

Mirror Mantra Beauty

Creating a new look for yourself can be a lot easier than you think, and it all starts with your eyebrows! First look at yourself lovingly in the mirror, and get as close as you can to your eyes to study them. Study the color, the layers, the light.

To create the lift in your eyes that many go to plastic surgeons for can be easily created with the perfect eyebrow arch. As you stare at your eyes, follow your gaze from the middle of the cornea up towards the center straight up to the brow. Measure from the cornea to the outer rim of the iris with your index finger or tweezers. The point of your arch should be in this radius. Now you can proceed to either tweeze a few of the hairs there yourself, or communicate to a trained brows professional that this is exactly where you want your arch to be.

While you're there staring at your beautiful windows of the soul remember to kindly say to yourself, "I love you and you are beautiful." Mirror work and affirmations can be a powerfully effective tool in creating a mental change within yourself and building confidence that will stay with you forever— as long as you're consistent! Start every morning before brushing your teeth with your mirror affirmations of love; and enjoy your new brows!

CHAPTER 4

Inner Eye Beauty

Wearing an eyebrow shape with a "fishhook" at the inner eye is one of the most common beauty mistakes that women make. The 'fishhook' brow makes the eyes appear much smaller and close together then they should. Recently when I was explaining to a client who was sporting the classic "fishhook" brow why it is wrong and how to correct it, I noticed that she wasn't really open to receiving my opinion and advice about her brows even though she'd asked.

Noticing that the fishhook brow she'd given herself was also giving her the appearance of having smaller eyes, I wondered if it was possible that, subconsciously, she wasn't as open-minded and receptive as she'd stated. As I continued to ponder this thought, I began to make the connection between eyes that are "closed down" with a mind that is closed down. I also began to think to myself that this woman might do well with some meditation tips. Generally, how we dress and wear our makeup and hair is intricately connected to how we are feeling on the inside; thus, the woman with the fishhook shape brow really isn't completely open to being her true self yet.

Shape your brows by tweezing away the hair at a 45-degree

angle throughout the end of the fishhook to create an open line for the brow. And when you're done, start a 15-minute daily practice of breathing with your eyes closed while imagining the color indigo at the spot between your two eyebrows. That focal point is called your third eye, and when it is open you will become more intuitive. An open third eye chakra will also help to allow you to truly see the beauty you are made of.

CHAPTER 5

Joy

It's the things that you do that create either joy or sadness. When you are doing something in life that makes you happy, it automatically triggers what I like to call the "happy hormones," serotonin and dopamine, to be released in the brain, assisting to stimulate positive feelings and excitement throughout the mind and body. This in turn creates a positive internal environment for improved health and wellbeing. If you are committed to creating a joyful life, then sticking to a hobby or career that makes you feel good is a sure and true sign that you are following your soul's divine path. Well done!

But let's say that this chosen career isn't providing you with an income, or not enough income? Believe me, I have a lot of experience in this area! So I know what I'm talking about when I say that your state of mind is everything in helping you to create, sustain, and live your life's true calling. Looking at the big picture is one thing, and knowing where you want to go and be is necessary, but it's the daily, baby steps that will take you there. Each and every day committing yourself to your joyful hobby or career, affirming what you want and not wavering from your conviction will help you achieve your goals. Ignore (or at least try to) the overnight success stories that you see in the media because that person may have had 500 lifetimes of struggling, and they may be getting their moment now. This about you and your joy!

Now let's say you are in a job that you hate, and you have a hobby you love. Many people experience this dilemma! I remember what my mother told me when I was at the beginning of my career and was totally broke! She said, "Well, doing what you love in life is half the battle. You're not like me, stuck in a job that you hate!"

Suppose you're in a job you hate because you need to support the family, and I'm telling you to do what you love! I know—how cliché and oh so spiritual! The truth is, nevertheless, that we're all here on this Earth for a reason, and the only way to find your own truth is by tuning into your own source and start listening for the truth. Meditation is one of the most basic and time-tested means for tuning in and listening. Yet in our busy and hectic society, many people have a resistance to meditation. In fact, I hear again and again from clients who are new to meditation, "I can't meditate!" I assure them, just as I wish to assure you, you can meditate. It simply requires commitment and follow-through.

Some of my happiest times of each and every day are when I sit quietly in the silence. The practice of meditation is quite like that of pursuing your dream career— it's all in the baby steps! Just start and commit to show up day after day, and your inner joy will begin to emerge. Because if you're not feeling it from the inside, you will never find true happiness on the outside.

CHAPTER 6

Taking Charge

One day you wake up and realize that your life isn't where you want it to be! You hem and haw about what to do! You get up, look in the mirror, and same reaction—more hemming and hawing! That's not the joyous sound of someone who is, perhaps not miserable, but not content either. Contentment with where you are in life and contentment with your body walk hand-in-hand! I could randomly ask 100 women if they are content with their career and body, and perhaps only one or two would actually say yes! Shocking, I know, but also quite true.

Feeling content on the inside and feeling content with how you look on the outside are intricately connected. Discontent can often result in being overweight, or the opposite can occur too, and a person develops an unhealthy obsession with exercise and thinness. So where and how do we find the balance?

I will be the first to admit that when I feel stressed and things are feeling a little out of my comfort zone, my gluten-free rule flies right out the door. Whether it's stress eating or over-exercising that gives you relief, these types of behaviors should signal an alarm in you that somewhere the balance between your mind and body is off. Luckily for me, at this point when things are riled up in my life, I've come far enough that I'm able to recognize the alarms and I'm able to quickly nip it in the bud. However, if you find that you are generally unhappy with your career, home life, or weight, then you've got to take charge and begin to take the steps towards your spiritual, mental, physical, and emotional stability.

It may feel overwhelming if you have 50 pounds to lose, or at the other end of the spectrum, perhaps it feels more difficult to get honest with yourself about how skinny you are. It starts with acknowledgement on the inside of you that you want to make changes, and that you are willing to take charge of your life and become your own leader!

Mental strength is the first step towards dedicating time every day to leading the life that you desire. Be honest with yourself and realistic at the same time. Start with writing down what you want. A list might look something like this:

Lose weight
Find a new job
Start my own business
Fall in love
Work on my marriage
Be a better mother

Whatever it is, start by writing it down. And be specific about what you want! An affirmation to attract the new job that you desire may go something like this: "It is now my intention to create an abundant income using my abilities and talents!" Retraining your brain may seem difficult, and it can take time, but nothing truly amazing happens overnight—at least not in my experience.

If you are at the point where you are not even sure of what you want, I assure you, you are not alone. Many people have gone to a place of such severe detachment that reconnecting to their dreams and goals can feel impossible. If this is you, then start by imagining the amazing energy that you are already made of, like on the cover of this book. You are a magnificent creative light that the world needs. By starting to acknowledge this within you, ideas will begin to percolate, and little by little, a clearer vision for your life will emerge. After you have begun to get comfortable with the idea that you are more than just a physical being, begin with this exercise every day. Commit to this practice for 30 days, and see what transpires in you and outside of you!

Begin by finding some quiet time and a space where you'll be uninterrupted.
Sit down in a comfortable position.
Breathe deeply and slowly in and out for 20 counts.
Imagine a deep blue color wave over you and focus it into the space between your eyes.
After the 20 breaths, rest here, breathing in the blue color.
Mentally state your affirmation, and slowly repeat it for 20 times while continuing to breathe.
If you have multiple affirmations, continue the steps for each one.

The most important action in taking charge of your life is taking charge of your mind. When beginning these techniques, it's equally as important to realize and believe that you are now connecting to your own source—the energy that you are made of. I recommend before starting this particular exercise that you have already begun the meditation practice first recommended on page one. The reason for this is that getting into the habit of taking time out to be still and acknowledge your great self is the foundational first step. Asking for what you want is second.

CHAPTER 7

Play

One of the most consistent mistakes that most of us make is that we work too hard. When we are in the pursuit of our dreams, we work very hard to achieve them, and what's left is very little time to play. We all have an inner child to attend to, and all too often neglect. My daughter said to me just yesterday that she wished she could have more play time in school! Human beings are naturally wired from birth and throughout childhood to live in a state of joy, to have fun, and create! It's in a child's natural state to desire this, and, of course, to receive love.

So why is it then that as we grow older we tend to forget that having fun is our human birthright? We feel guilty about playing hooky and heading to a movie. Seriously, when was the last time you went to the park and took a simple ride on the swing set? Do it and see how much joy it brings, and how much fun it is to feel like a kid again! One of my favorite things to do for fun is to go sledding with my daughter. Getting on the sled and barreling down the hill, screaming all the way down brings me right back to my childhood, which feels amazing.

When we are stuck in life or feeling depressed, tending to our inner child and having a bit of fun is exactly what we should do. "What is my inner child?" you might be asking. Our inner child is the purest part of our being that lies closely within our hearts and memories— kind of like a first love. It is the essential part of our spirit that remains uncluttered and free.

Sometimes due to trauma in childhood, your inner child can be hurt. When this occurs, you, as an adult, must take steps to nurture this part of yourself so you can live a free life filled with all the love you deserve. Your inner child represents the purity of your spirit and when it is consistently nurtured you will begin to exude an energy that people will automatically be drawn to—quite similarly as to when you are drawn to the innocence of a child or baby.

So whatever it is that you love to do for fun, start by making the commitment to do this for yourself on a regular basis, as long as it doesn't include an excessive amount of alcohol, eating, or shopping! When you give yourself the chance to laugh, be joyous, and play you will energetically unblock the things in your life that aren't working because you are giving your life force an opportunity to flow freely through your mind, body, and spirit.

CHAPTER 8

Moderation

As I talk about the importance of practicing meditation throughout the pages of this book, it's equally important to accept the principle of moderation in your life too. Excess food, alcohol, technology, social media, television, and the news, to name just a few, suggest all too clearly that excess runs rampant in our lives. Living more simplistically can clear the way to finding what we are truly searching. Cutting back on excess in our lives opens our energy fields and homes to receiving what matters most for our soul's highest purpose in life.

Do you really need to live in a mansion? To own several designer bags? To wear fake hair and eyelashes? If you are completely honest with yourself, and sincerely intend to feel your beauty from the inside out, you will not hesitate to ask yourself these questions and to be honest with your answers. I'm not saying it's wrong to have nice things because I like nice things too. However, I do not have an excess of "stuff" in my life because I realized a long time ago that I don't need it to feel happy or important!

Practicing moderation in all areas of your life is a crucial step to realizing your full potential in becoming aligned with your source of energetic beauty. Having too much stuff and extravagance is distracting from what truly matters and keeps us from feeling the purest forms of compassion and love for all of humanity.

Let me give you an example of what I'm talking about! When I was a young girl just beginning my career, I moved to Italy to further pursue my dreams of building a career as an artist. I will never forget how it seemed to me at the time that practically everyone I noticed seemed to be wearing expensive designer clothing from head-to-toe. I was simultaneously impressed and intimidated, as I had nothing of the sort to wear, and I was often the focus of many an unwanted stare.

After some time had passed, I asked a very wise Italian friend how it was that everyone was rich, and where were all the poor people like me? He laughed and responded, "Oh, my dear, they may be wearing Armani on the outside, but it's more than likely that they have no furniture in their homes!" Aha! The light bulb went off, and I got it! They were dressing to impress, and hadn't a lira after all!

Presenting a false illusion of yourself through excess and extravagance will not bring you real happiness at all; merely a false sense of self, and a whole lot of insecurity! Creating a sense of more compassion and self-love will help you take baby steps to begin to take stock of what you really need and really do not. Then take an honest look at yourself in the mirror. Get your head out of the clouds, and ask yourself what you need to let go of that is excessive in your life. For example, do you really need hair extensions? Do you really need to wear makeup every day?

Playing with your hair, makeup, and wardrobe, and enjoying creating looks is one thing, but being dependent upon outer beauty and fashion tools is another thing altogether. Make a commitment to be hair and makeup-clean one day every week, and begin to get comfortable with your unadulterated appearance and self. And while you're at it, go ahead and donate one of your designer bags to someone who doesn't have any! Moderation is the key to becoming more self-aware, and giving is the next step to true beauty from the inside out.

CHAPTER 9

Persistence

Do you find yourself in the midst of turmoil and hectic happenings in your life, causing you to get your feathers in a tussle? Are unexpected problems, situations, or people popping into your life and creating chaos? Did you know that, subconsciously, we attract these messes into our lives as a way to work through old patterns that we haven't yet fully learned from and released? Even if these things are lessons, we can get utterly annoyed because we have to get things done, we want the perfect life, and these problems are getting in our way!

Believe me, I am not immune. My entire life has been filled with one learning experience after another, prompting me to consciously continue study, reflect, and participate fully in my own life and evolution with great persistence. Persistence in creating the life, look, and feel you want out of life comes from exactly that—being persistent! Nothing just happens without some sort of cosmic interaction in life. The universe just doesn't work that way.

Let say, for example, that you keep attracting long-distance relationships. Over and over, love comes with a plane ticket and travel over the ocean! You ask yourself, "Why can't I just find someone who lives here?" But the truth is, subconsciously, you don't really want authentic intimacy; and wearing love on your sleeve suits your conscious mind better than dealing with your subconscious mind because that's just too much work! In reality, these subconsciously created problems are bringing patterns into your conscious awareness to show you that there is indeed an imbalance. Moreover, the imbalance is one that you have the power to correct.

Persistent problems are actually insistent reminders that this is something your soul wants you to acknowledge, work on, and release! So how do we do this? Acknowledgment is the first step. Then with persistence in meditation, exercise, affirmations, prayer, cleansing, and good old fun, you can begin to recreate new patterns. As you do this, the old problems will eventually dissipate.

Start with a daily ritual that will help to relax your mind and body, like taking a simple sea salt and lavender bath. Sea salt helps detox and cleanse the body, while lavender calms the senses.

Persistently creating an atmosphere in your life and circumstances that is calming and nurturing will help you to gently become more aware of negative patterns. In turn, you'll open yourself up to possibilities for positive change.

CHAPTER 10

Debauchery

It's a fact that when you have a hangover, you're more likely to overindulge the next day with carbs, fat, sugar, and even more alcohol! Debauchery! We've all been there.

Why do we overindulge, go nuts, and lose control? The answer is simple, yet may be difficult to understand or accept. When we are detached from our inner harmony, we look for ways to escape. Oftentimes, escaping from our inner turmoil is the easiest way to heal ourselves—or so we think.

We take vacations to get away from stress, but I so often hear people say after they return from their vacation, that it was actually stressful! Hmmm... So then we need another way to de-stress and escape! It becomes cyclical, this need to get away from ourselves. When you commit to getting comfortable with your real vibration through meditation, for example, the number of evenings of getting drunk will start to lessen, the food binges will diminish, and smoking will come to an end.

Creating positive change in your life can feel hard at first because it challenges your will to be completely conscious, which means your ego is no longer the center of your attention. This also means that the things that are not good for you—and this can include people too—become uncomfortable for you; and it can be difficult to let things or people go.

When you take the first step in beginning your meditation practice, an effective mantra and affirmation to use on a frequent basis to help ease the discomfort of transition is this: "Dear God, please deliver me from all that no longer serves my highest and greatest good, and give me the strength to stay true to my heart and beautiful self."

CHAPTER 11

Highlighting

Are you feeling bright and light in your heels one day, and heavy and fat the next? A common problem amongst today's modern woman! We alter our mood according to the external influences occurring in our lives at any given time. When something great happens, it gives us that pep in our step, and we shine a little brighter for a period of time.

As a society we have become far too attached to the external side of ourselves. As our attachment to the external grows, we connect our happiness with outer influences, circumstances, and, yes, to our looks. As we falsely connect our happiness with external influences it can strengthen our desire to head to the salon for a new round of highlights far too frequently. It's also true that we do the same thing when we are feeling depressed—we head to the salon for some highlights, thinking that it will help us feel better.

Whether we are happy and sad, external beauty therapy becomes the inextricable thing that supports our emotions and feels like something we can always count on. We use external beauty tools to subconsciously express how we are feeling on the inside.

For instance, I have always had dark brown hair, but I remember a time when I was living in Los Angeles that all of a sudden I developed a desire for red hair! I did everything I could to get the perfect shade of red, and I wasn't satisfied for months until I got it!

One day I met with a wise, old friend who'd not seen me in a while. He commented, "You must be going through a transformative time out here in L.A, expressing yourself by changing your hair color!" WHAT? I hadn't a clue what he meant. However, later when I had looked back on that time in my life, I distinctly remember that I was very lonely and I was chasing a guy who didn't know that I existed, thus resulting in my determination for red hair and the subconscious need to fill a void in my life that I wasn't filling with my own spirit. What I learned is that when you are experiencing any extreme emotion or action in your life that brings upon a need to dramatically alter your appearance, that's exactly when, in fact, you shouldn't run straight to the salon!

Instead, take some time to account for the way you are feeling, and acknowledge your loneliness, pain and even your joy. Ask yourself if you're heading to the salon to treat yourself (which is perfectly ok), or are you heading there because you think if you change your hair color it will make your life better in some way?

Beauty therapy in all its splendor can be a glorious way to express your creativity, but it shouldn't be used as way to hide unresolved emotions that need to be healed. If after reflection you come to the conclusion that indeed getting a few highlights is truly an uncluttered and beautiful expression of yourself at this moment in time, then by all means go for it! And while you're there make sure to tell your stylist that you want highlights that best complement your skin tone and eyes, a shade that will highlight the already beautiful you!

CHAPTER 12

Magnificent

You are MAGNIFICENT! Realizing this can take some time and commitment to yourself, and what makes that challenging is that far too often we don't prioritize self-care. Especially if you're a mother like I am, you tend to cater to everyone else's needs before your own, and then feel guilty if you take time for yourself. I have found that much like starting a new diet, the commitment begins to fall by the way side when life gets crazy. Along with your new diet, your self-care routine flies out the door. Feeling that detachment from self, old insecurities, binging habits, or excessive highlights start all over again.

Like when our baby starts to take their first steps and realizes for the first time they have legs that can do this, they commit fully with their subconscious and conscious mind, as if to say, "by God, I'm going to walk!" That's what it takes each and every day—baby steps and a fierce desire with your subconscious and conscious mind to commit to the MAGNIFICENT you. The you that is light, power, creation, and love.

The ego and our busy lives and others' demands want us to be ramped up with stress and despair, and shutters at the prospect of us unleashing our magnificent selves. But what do you truly want? To fall back and forth between 20 unwanted pounds, an unhappy love life, and job you hate, or living the life you were meant to live? Much like making the intention to start a new cleanse or diet, so should be the choice to do something that constitutes absolute self-care.

Everything in your life is a direct reflection of what's going on inside of you, so that is why dedication to self-care is essential to your overall wellbeing and ultimate beauty. Whether it's yoga classes, pedicures, or reflexology and massage treatments take the time to commit to taking care of you, to nourish your inner beauty so your outer beauty can shine like never before.

CHAPTER 13

Acceptance

We are in judgment! Of ourselves, and admit it, of everyone else too. Even when we try to practice non-judgment of others, it's incredibly difficult to do. On the subway here in New York just the other day, there was a man sitting across from me having an entire, hot meal of Chinese food in his seat. He was chowing down and not the least bit concerned about anyone around him. My eye settled right in on him and I caught a terrible staring attack!

As the smell of the food permeated the entire subway car I began to get annoyed, and then it started—"the judgment!" I mean, how could I not? I began to look at him and wonder how he could have such a lack of respect for the rest of us on this train. He was oblivious to the smell of the food and that it was irritating me beyond belief. I shamefully thought to myself that he had absolutely no manners whatsoever, and how uncouth to eat so "slobberishly" like that in public!

However, through all my learning I soon started to realize that judging him was wrong! Perhaps he had been working all night and was heading to a day job and this was his only opportunity to eat. I soon began to re-center my focus on him and shift it to that of positive feelings. It was hard! I started to breathe in and out gently while positively affirming to myself and silently to him that "the God in me salutes the God in you!" Over and over I mentally repeated this affirmation while calmly continuing to breathe. He finished eating, got his things in order, and then suddenly looked up and caught my eye and gently smiled. I returned the smile and relaxed, mentally apologizing for judging him so harshly.

When we impose negative thoughts on others we energetically are giving that energy right back to ourselves. Ever heard of bad karma? The law of attraction? All is created through loving or negative thoughts. Being in a place of absolute non-judgment all of the time was something that Jesus achieved!

Me and you? We've got to nip it in the bud as soon as we feel it creeping up so that we too can move towards greater tolerance of our fellow man and realize our own power and light like Jesus did. Living in the knowing that we are all truly one, and accepting each other's differences, behaviors, looks and beliefs is all part of our learning process here on Earth. So the next time you honestly feel as if you are placing judgment on someone else, know that you are not helping anyone, least of all yourself.

Take a moment to breathe and affirm, "Today I will be in non-judgment."

CHAPTER 14

Beauty Rules

Long hair, short hair, red lip, pale lip! What to do with our look has become the "it" thing. Especially in the last few years, the social media phenomenon has further expanded the broad reach of the very powerful and influential beauty industry. Taking good care of our health and bodies is of invaluable necessity, and sometimes that leads to an automatic desire to further enhance our outer beauty by tweaking our appearance with external beauty tools, in the way we wear our hair, makeup, and clothing. It is simply called self-respect, which in turn equals self-care, which in then turn leads to self-empowerment!

The problem with external beauty tools is that, as I've mentioned before, they can trick us into believing they will solve our problems, relieve our sadness and depression, or clear away blockages in general. Going to extremes and losing awareness of what is truly excessive and what is not is when we need to take stock and look internally at what's really going on. Following the latest beauty trend is something that I don't usually counsel women to do because beauty companies that have products to sell create the so-called trends.

So how do you find the best look for you and which tools to

use that will easily help you accentuate your own unique beauty? I always tell a client they have to become their own beauty expert in some respects, to learn to feel it. When you want to try out a look, and you've been doing the inner work through meditation, you will intuitively be drawn to colors and hairstyles that will work best with your features.

Rather than following a strict set of beauty rules, like the old rule of not wearing long hair after 40, for example, which is utterly ridiculous, let the new wave of expression for women be that of pure and utter joy! Joy in creating your own definitive beauty from deep within that resonates throughout your entire being through the ether and to the ends of your eyelashes, lips and hair color too.

Here's a new beauty rule for women: when in doubt about how or what to do with your hair and makeup, pause and breathe. Allow yourself to feel a sense of joy on the inside. Then, from a place of calm balance, become your own best expert and go have fun!

CHAPTER 15

Love

The famous tune comes to mind as I think about love! Come on, sing it with me, "All you need is love, all you need is love, all you need is love, love, love is all you need!"

We all need love to prosper, thrive, and, quite frankly, stay alive! We look for it online, at the gym, or, the old fashioned way, in a bar. We desire a love relationship to feel complete and to flourish within ourselves. Still, through all the time spent searching for love, many people stay single or in relationships that are highly dysfunctional, or find themselves "falling" in and out of love. It can be a challenge to be alone and truly love, honor, and enjoy your own company without the need for a romantic relationship.

I am not a relationship expert! However, I did get a few things right along my journey in finding love.

1. I maintained a consistent devotion to my meditation and spiritual practice.
2. I never ever was attracted to the same type of guy over and over!

3. I was open to receiving love! When my husband arrived into my life he wasn't at all what I was expecting, but love came in a soul that knew mine and I knew his!

My point is this—when you have a preconceived conviction of what type of person will make you happy, you will never find soul love. It's a fact!

"He's not my type" or "I'm not attracted to him!" I've heard it repeatedly over the years from various people, all still single! Finding love starts with you and you alone. You have to love the real you and devote time every day to becoming acquainted with your source, because once it is truly unleashed from within, you will begin to attract in different types of people that before you would never have considered or been drawn to.

Start simply by asking your source to come forth with love in quiet time every day. I always begin my meditation with these words:

"Dear God, I ask with love that you be with me now." Begin your breathing deeply in and out, focusing on your heart center. It is in the silence that the love we are made of shines through from the inside out. Basking in this love, before you know it, five minutes of meditation will quickly turn into 30.

Surround yourself with things that make you feel loved, like fresh flowers in your home every week. Make yourself up for you and you alone, if that's what makes you feel good. Ultimately, when you love yourself totally, love will come, and the key to recognizing a soul love comes from an awareness awakened from deep within.

CHAPTER 16

The Plastic Veil

I will never get any form of plastic surgery! That said, I fully admit that I was unhappy with my looks and felt insecure about myself when I was younger. In fact, when I was in my early 20's, I was so insecure that I attracted a boyfriend who used to constantly tell me that I was fat and that his preferred type of woman was a skinny blonde! I attracted in a partner who felt the same about me that I did about myself.

I didn't realize at the time what was going on, but I was conscious enough to know that what he was doing was abusive, and I eventually left. A common plague amongst younger women today is to feel bad on the inside while looking great on the outside, which equals a dysfunctional relationship with themselves and in their love relationships. I've worked with hundreds of beautiful models over the years—perhaps even thousands—and many subconsciously wanted to tell me about their life and what was going on. I soon realized that even though I was not model-skinny or airbrush-pretty, these girls had exactly the same problems that I did: dysfunctional partners and lives!

The essence of a woman is pure beauty. Pure beauty is not

body-centric and focused on being skinny or outwardly pretty. The confidence and joy that a woman exudes is the purest form of beauty. As I've reached my mid-forties, I keep hearing from many that I haven't aged, and look great and asked what my secret is.

Well, I distinctly recall that when I started my daily meditation practice, many people were telling me how amazing I looked and asking what I doing. Was it a new diet? Was I in love? Was it my day cream? It went on and on. The only thing that had changed was that I'd started tuning into myself consistently, everyday through mindful meditation. The glow was coming from inside of me, not from any other source or beauty tool.

So here I am telling you that the greatest anti-aging secret is pure and simple; that's my experience and it's what I really believe. I'm not saying I don't use beauty creams and remedies—I do. But I keep my regimen simple and use pure ingredients to support my skin and elasticity.

I've consistently found that a woman who's had plastic surgery of any kind looks unlike their best self. Often, the surgical changes actually make a person look older, and can be a sign that there's something off on the inside. Holding onto youth should be something that is honored by identifying with your inner child and having fun. It shouldn't be to continue to try to look as young as you possibly can with the help of a scalpel. Lifting eyelids and falsely erasing wrinkles is denying the opportunity to feel the real you and embrace the present.

If you feel the pressure is immense to have bigger eyes or a flat stomach, first ask yourself with a quiet and gentle mind if this is the truth for you. Could there be another path to feeling happy with yourself? The answer is, of course, there is. I'm living proof that tuning into your source is the pudding you really need.

CHAPTER 17

Hope

Hope is a word that pretty much defined most of my entire young adulthood in some way or another. I hope I get that job! I hope I get that guy! I hope someone buys a painting! I hope I get that apartment.

Merriam-Webster's online definition of hope is "to cherish a desire with anticipation."[1] Having the desire and hope for an occurrence that you propose through your own free will that you are certain will bring you relief, joy, and even excitement is wonderful as long as it's aligned with your source.

Hopelessness—now that's another story, and the two, hopelessness and hope, are so closely intertwined that oftentimes they can occur at the same time. What do I mean by that? Well, here is an example.

A few years back I was actively pitching my first television pilot of "Morning Moms." I was full of hope! At the same time, with each and every rejection, hopelessness crept up on me and left me with a feeling of despair. I remember at the end of my pitch season and getting a contract on the table ready to be signed, that I had a feeling of great excitement (i.e. hope), and at the same time I was worried

[1] *Merriam Webster Online*, Retrieved April 3, 2016, from https://www.merriam webster.com/dictionary/hope.

something would go wrong because I had already endured so much rejection (i.e. hopelessness). Right before we were to sign the deal, the producer changed his mind at the last minute and decided not to take a chance on me. He said he didn't think I had enough passion for the project, even though I was the creator!

I was filled with hopelessness about myself, my abilities and, quite frankly, I was in doubt about every area of my life at that point. I had given all of my energy, time, and money to my project just to have it deflated by someone's judgment in a split second. However, after some time had passed, I began to shake it off and redirect my focus.

Hopelessness turned itself back into hope once again, but this time hope blossomed not because I was attached to something that was about to happen or that I wanted to happen. It was inside me after I'd redirected my focus to healing myself from hopelessness and disappointment. My meditation practice helped me regain my composure and sense of self after what I'd considered a major setback in my career and life. Because, you see, as I was filled with so much hope that I was finally going to get my big break, during that time I had let my meditation practice fall by the wayside.

What I learned is this: when we are full of hope that's attached to a specific outcome because we believe that outcome will somehow complete us, that's a mistake. Because I was filled with hope and hopelessness at the same time, the universe gave me exactly that—an almost TV show! My dream was incomplete because my hope was tainted by hopelessness.

When we affirm to our source that we want our work to be lifted to its highest possibility in life, we then align with our soul's divine path and our hopes, dreams, and goals will never bring us a feeling of hopelessness because they are our divine right and occur in the divine time of things. So when you are in a whirlpool of despair and your hope starts to make you nervous, take a step back and retreat into the quiet, and ask that your hopelessness gets replenished with divine love; and the truth for you and your life's mission and purpose will be revealed!

CHAPTER 18

Confidence

Confidence. Where does it come from, who has it, and how do we get it? Like soul love, it cannot be bought! Insecurity and confidence are frequently disguised in each other and oftentimes both hide our true selves. We usually feel the most confident about ourselves when things are going well in our life. Your career is great! Great partner! Happy marriage! It puts the sync into our lives and when things seem to be going well for an extended period of time, then woo hoo! You haven't had to deal with one internal thing.

I remember when the stock market crashed in 2008, I knew many people who lost a lot of money, as well as their jobs. Freak out time came on a collective level! I knew that even though there was a trickledown effect, it needed to happen because when we are riding life's highest waves—those based solely on aesthetics and wealth acquisition—it can't and won't continue forever, materially nor energetically.

When something happens to trigger feelings of despair, that despair time and again leads to insecurity, and then all too often a familiar pity party begins, and we wonder "why me?" Negativity ensues and all the other stuff you've been suppressing riles itself up, and BAM! Self-confidence flies out the door, and so goes the plummet into self-deprecation.

Rather than associate confidence with external influences, we have to redirect our attention onto the eternal power that lives within us so that when sudden change occurs and our outer circumstances are thrust into turmoil, we are not pushed to fight and ward off depression and anxiety. Instead, we take calm-minded steps, breathe deeply, and know that there is always something to learn, and that each phase of external circumstances is really just a temporary call from your source to take a closer look at your life, to learn and grow.

Just imagine a world where meditation and the focus of upliftment of consciousness was the norm for everyone. There would be less corruption on Wall Street, terrorism wouldn't be in the nightly news, and we would see the light magnificently shining through all those we encounter.

So the next time you tell yourself you're not good enough and your confidence is lost, stop and bring yourself back to center where rebalancing can happen. Affirm these truths:

I am powerful!
I am beauty.
I am intelligence.
I am love.
I am magnificent!
I am compassion.

Let your inner goddess power you through all circumstances, good and bad, because if you do, you will rarely feel insecure again.

CHAPTER 19

Duality

The beauty in you and outside of you is circumstantial if you are unable to balance both your masculine and feminine energies. For example, let's say that you are addicted to wearing high heels and pink lipstick every day, you only do yoga, and you manage a flower shop! Wonderful! But here's the thing—we are all made up of both masculine and feminine energies and it's important to acknowledge and become comfortable with the non-dominant side of ourselves so we can then fully enjoy beautiful balance from the inside out.

My seven-year daughter is a total girly-girl! She loves her dolls, her clothes, and loves to play with hair and makeup. With her father, however, her favorite thing to do on a daily basis is to play karate and wrestle. She's as fully at home in her body wearing pretty pink as she is throwing a powerful karate chop; hence she presents an equalized balance between her feminine and masculine sides.

If children are brought up in a balanced and loving home and nurtured from soul love, then their natural attunement with their source is clearer and less uninterrupted than most adults, resulting in the masculine and feminine energies being naturally aligned. Imbalance starts to occur as we grow older, as outer influences begin to steer us off our true energetic path of self-love and beauty. Peer pressure, media, and magazines all have a powerful ability to lure humanity away from our own pure, loving selves; and the ego continues to dominate the world. How do we recognize and align our masculine and feminine energies? Start with a checklist of questions like these.

1. Do you constantly give to others and feel uncomfortable and guilty receiving help and love?
2. Are you attracted to partners that are controlling and domineering?
3. Are you uncomfortable going out the door without your makeup on?

If you answered yes to any of these questions, then you are enabling your feminine self to be more dominant in your life, and a good kickboxing class might be in order! If you are enabling your masculine self to be more dominant, then you may be someone who wouldn't be caught dead with a stitch of makeup on, or you prefer wearing masculine clothes. Or you attract partners with whom you can easily and always get your way.

Because humanity is so closely connected and attached to how we express ourselves through our appearance as a result from being severely detached from source, an evident indicator of your feminine and masculine energies being in a state of imbalance can be easily identified in how you present yourself on the outside and in your relationships and friendships. The key to balancing your duality is by allowing both sides to be expressed freely from time to time. For example, if you are the woman who runs the flower shop and only does yoga, switch up your routine and try a kickboxing class once in a while. And if you are the woman who hates to wear makeup, go for it, and unleash your inner diva with a fabulous cat eye!

We are complex human beings, full of energy. Channeling it all in the same direction can muddle the divine flow within you, which can lead to an inauthentic representation of your truest beauty.

CHAPTER 20

Exercise

Exercising your body is essential to your overall physical and mental wellbeing. Many people thrive on daily physical routines. The young and the beautiful are working out to stay thin and look their best. But how many exercise enthusiasts pay as much attention to their meditation practice? I can't tell you how many people I've worked with who are pretty much their own workout expert. I've been advised by practically all of New York for the last 20 years, so I know a lot about, yoga, Pilates, running, weight training, and on and on! What I have to come to realize, however, is that most of the people who are regimented about their workouts and physical selves, aren't so much about their spiritual selves.

The reason I talk about the importance of meditating on a daily basis is because when you are tuned in and fully capable of listening to your own source, it will no longer be necessary to head to the gym every day, or to use exercise as a tool to falsely manipulate your belief system about your feelings and looks. I'm not saying don't exercise or that it isn't important. It is, but when you are living consciously from the inside out, exercise becomes another way to release stagnant energy, boost your physical immune system, and enhance your mental brain function, which is important for your lifelong health.

The physical body is our temple, which hosts our source; so when we tune in on a daily basis our source will tell us which exercise will best uplift our health for that time frame. Your workouts will begin to take on a different feeling of completion and satisfaction. You will no longer run to the mirror or get on the scale afterwards.

Because exercise is meant to compliment and support our spiritual development, it isn't meant to solely control our external appearance. When you are aligned with your source your weight will naturally stay in the same range for long periods of time. You will no longer desire to binge excessively or feel guilty about not making it to the gym. The world needs to exercise their spirit a lot more first, and then get moving! Because by exercising your spirit first, you'll feel the lightness you are made of, and the physical exercise then becomes a tool to further support and nourish your overall wellbeing, which in turn will help you achieve the beauty you desire for the world to see.

CHAPTER 21

Mother Earth

Walking through a majestic garden filled with glorious flowers and plants; walking along a beach with a mesmerizing sunset and hearing the sound of soothing waves breaking on the shore; hiking in the mountains and observing the stunning rock formations, all ways of listening to the nurturing voice of Mother Earth.

Being at one with nature and our beautiful planet is an intoxicating and peaceful place to be. If you are lucky enough to be, or if divine planning has placed you, in a location on Earth where you live in one of these beautiful settings, then you may find it easier to relax and connect with nature. But if you are like me, and your circumstances and subconscious desires have you in a huge metropolis like New York City, then it is not logically in the daily cards to take a walk up into the mountains or stroll along a tropical beach. It's winter here now as I write, and the cold chills to the bone. It's hard to get out for long periods of time, and even a walk over to Central Park can feel daunting. So what to do?

Connecting with nature and allowing the vibration of pure, unequivocal, and natural beauty to run through your mind and body is essential to our spiritual, mental, and physical wellbeing and promotes an undeniable appeal to our appearance. I use my meditation practice to tune into nature and connect with Mother Earth by meditating upon an image like a tropical paradise and a calming ocean to help me balance the lack of outdoor time. Essential oils and incense can also assist you when you find connecting directly to nature isn't right at your fingertips.

The other day as I briskly walked along the city sidewalks, anxious to get to my destination to escape -10 degrees, I was struck by the clear, blue sky and blazing rays of sunshine. As I approached a crosswalk, the light changed and I distinctly and immediately felt soothed by the sunlight on my face. I closed my eyes and deeply, quietly breathed the sun in and out. I fell into a place of absolute peace and comfort, allowing the power of Mother Earth to connect with me even on a busy, loud, and freezing corner of New York. I missed the light change and continued to stay for another few moments on my mini-meditation-vacation, feeling warm, calm and refreshed.

Mother Earth and nature are here to support our journey in this lifetime, to help us fully embrace our true beauty and selves. She is like you—naturally powerful, majestic, and beautiful. And, like you, she needs care, time, love, and respect.

When you can begin to take time to connect with Mother Earth and adopt her strength, power, and magnificence as an important part of your beauty regime, you'll then begin to see that she already lives within you, and that the connection is just waiting to be healed and nourished. Much like a houseplant requires water and light to stay alive, so does your soul. Use the power of the sun or a ray of light to recharge your connection to Mother Earth. Call her forth and acknowledge her, embrace her, and love her no matter the time of year or location you are in.

CHAPTER 22

Ego and Depression

No one is immune from depression, and dark days come upon each of us at some time in life. For some, it comes in frequent spells; for others, once in a blue moon; and for the others still, it lives and breathes in their lives on a daily basis. Medication has become a readily handed Band-Aid for many who work in, or rely on, the medical field. As a collective, there is a powerful belief that medication is the only remedy for certain chemical imbalances.

It's true, for example, that particularly in women, hormonal fluctuations can have an impact on their mental health and wellbeing. However, for these natural occurrences, holistic remedies, such as nutrition, exercise, and meditation can assist in supporting mood swings and occasional depression.

I remember when Brook Shields and Tom Cruise were in the media, hashing out the use of medication for women with postpartum depression. I fully admit that I too had a terrible case of "the baby blues" after I had my daughter, but because I'd already developed a meditation practice, I used breastfeeding time to simultaneously feed my child and meditate. Meditation was a natural source of medication, balance, and soul-bonding for both of us. I can honestly say that without it, I never would have made it through that period of my life. So I'm not judging Brook Shields or anyone else who needs medication as a supportive tool for helping with chemical imbalances. But what I am saying is that if you fully commit to a deep and fulfilling meditation and spiritual practice, you'll less likely need medication to be the primary support tool.

Depression takes lives! It doesn't have to be that way, but sadly when there is a severe detachment from source within the conscious mind, the ego will dominate your thoughts and feelings to create a consistent feeling of doom and gloom. However, when you consistently connect to your source through meditation, you enable the light and the most powerful part of you to be predominant in your subconscious and conscious mind, which creates an environment of peace and mental stability. When you are detached from your source, which is God flowing through you, the ego or dark energy predominates, and this is when mental instability can grow and become more dominant in your conscious mind.

When we witness someone in the public eye, for example, commit suicide as a result of depression, it shocks us and we all ask what they could've possibly be so depressed about. They are famous, rich, have a gorgeous family, and are mega-talented—they have it all! Or so we think. Here's what I know and have witnessed firsthand: the bigger your life's mission and soul purpose, the more the ego will fight you, possibly resulting in depression on a grander scale!

Being famous and having extreme material wealth is where the ego thrives. So if you haven't done the inner work, or aren't doing any at all, and are detached from your source, then substance abuse will thrive, relationships will continue to fail, and a complex and inaccurate sense of self will dominate your life, resulting in the inevitable depression.

Or, perhaps on the other hand, you are stuck in a job you hate, or you are unemployed and flat broke. But unbeknownst to you, your soul's highest purpose could be to write a book that will uplift the world on a distinctive level and will be around for hundreds of years for others to read and learn from! Your logical mind can't comprehend this though because you failed 12th grade English and the thought of writing a book is so overwhelming, seemingly preposterous, and downright terrifying that it literally blocks you from doing what you are meant to be doing in this life. A set of circumstances and childhood beliefs about yourself and the ego set you in opposition to your soul's quest.

Nonetheless, your source is more powerful than your ego, so by giving yourself the attention you truly need, the writer in you will be born! It's undeniable that when you support your source and allow the beauty you're made of to shine through, your soul's purpose will begin to fall into place. I know that naysayers and critics might say, "She's crazy, she's claiming that meditation is the key to curing depression."

I'm not saying that exactly, but meditation can and will support an upliftment of consciousness, which in turn leads to a stronger connection to your source. And when you allow source to take over a depressing day by letting go and getting in that great, 30-minute meditation session, it will shift your day, mood, and chemical neurons within the body away from what was bringing you down in the first place.

CHAPTER 23

Contouring

Sharp edges and rounded curves take form in various ways in our lives and in our looks. We set up structure in our daily lives in the form of schedules, appointments, and calorie counting. We also contour our lips, cheeks, nose, and chin to keep our looks in check with the current, acceptable trends.

If things are too rigid in your life, you may be like the person who can't function in an atmosphere that isn't meticulously clean, for example. You literally can't sleep at night knowing that there is a speck of dust on the dining table, and you obsess over minute details that take up your time, creating unwanted stress. You may suffer from high blood pressure or Irritable Bowel Syndrome.

Or you could be someone who is a complete slob and doesn't care at all about cleanliness, and are not even aware that your house is dirty! You may have Type 2 diabetes and suffer from chronic headaches.

Many experts find it appropriate to label personality types. For example, if you are like the woman who is obsessed with cleaning, you have a type-A personality. Whether it is scientifically proven or not, I've always found the labeling and categorizing of people by types to be extremely odd. This may be because I could never completely find myself in any of the types; I've always felt like I'm a combination of types all at the same time. Spiritually speaking, of course, it's impossible to label someone a type because all souls are created equal. It is in the outer conditioning and belief systems that sharpen the edges of someone's spirit and rounds the corners of their desires and intentions.

So perhaps personality type-A could become more like a combination of all the types if more attention was placed upon the soul's nourishment. What I mean is, everything we do and wear is according to some lifelong conditioning that has a powerful pull on how we live, unless we've already incorporated some spiritual meaning into life. False beliefs or patterns can be so deeply etched into our existence that it affects our life patterns and outcomes, even when we try to change and set new goals. The curves and edges we have subconsciously set up stand so tall that they feel like a fierce mountain before us that we're convinced we could never climb.

So how do we soften the edges and straighten the corners of our lives that don't seem to be working? I suggest to first stop labeling yourself in any way, like, "I'm too skinny" or "I'm too fat." You are a beautiful soul first and foremost and labels and stereotypes that are provided by society aren't helping anyone at all. To judge yourself solely by a mind deeply rooted in your subconscious conditioning, or even worse, by the media, isn't uplifting your state of consciousness in any way, shape, or form.

The only one who should shape you is your higher self. It takes time and gentle care to paint your life softly and beautifully the way it was intended by source. Too much or too little self-control are obvious indicators that we need to either loosen or tighten the grip that we have on our lives, whether through too much action or no action at all. The polarities signify detachment, and a little more flexibility can help you infuse more balance and more character into your personality type.

So manicure and contour your home and looks much the same way you would tend to a lovely garden with care, nourishment, appreciation, love, and time, and begin to see that you will no longer be able to define yourself by a strict set of personality rules and stereotypes.

Chapter 24

Color Therapy

Imagine a world where the sky is always infused with the most majestic purples and oranges, the trees are filled with vibrant indigo blues, and the color around you is infinite and ever-changing. If you focus for a moment on the cover of this book, you will see an exhilarating spiritual beauty filled with colorful energy, who can morph her vibration from one series of colors to another. You are that beauty! So just imagine that within you and around you is an invisible aura of color that reflects and responds to your human emotions and will.

I was introduced to auras back in the early 90's when I first had an aura photo taken of me. It took me by surprise and delighted me at the same time to see and realize that I was made up of more than just my fears and the feeling of weight in my body. Thus began my journey into spiritual exploration and renewal in this life.

When I started painting back then, it quickly became apparent the ability of Spirit to produce and present energy through a brilliant array of colors. As an artist, I have an ability to tap into a creative source that is beyond my own human consciousness. When I tune into my source, I am able to allow a flow of energetic color and information to be produced—much like the writing of this book.

As we become more evolved in our meditation practice and develop our energetic senses, we then further enable our ability to connect with color as a tool to heal and glow from the inside out. For example, I live in New York City, and black is a color that is predominantly featured in fashion as well as on the street. Black does not enable the vibration of the soul to pulsate at its highest potential. It diminishes it. I'm not saying that I never wear black because I do if it looks good in an outfit. But if I'm feeling down for any reason, I will never choose to wear black. Because I'm more acutely sensitive to the power of color vibrations, I won't wear black when I need extra support during a bad day. That goes for the colors I choose for my makeup as well.

Vibrant colors such as purple, indigo blue, emerald green, and gold are fabulous colors to have in your wardrobe and in your makeup palette to support your inner spirit and outer aura. I have a silk green and blue scarf that I frequently wear around my neck for two reasons:

(1) I love it, and (2) green and blue are the colors that enhance the throat and heart chakras, which support love, communication, truth, and integrity, characteristics that are required to live in alignment with your best and most authentic self. To more clearly understand which colors will best support your inner radiance, begin by incorporating colors that are aligned with the chakras of your body into your meditation practice by visualizing them flowing in and out with the rhythm of your breathing.

1. Root chakra is located at the tailbone and spine (red).
2. Sacral chakra is located in the lower abdomen (orange).
3. Solar Plexus chakra is located in the upper abdomen (yellow).
4. Heart chakra is located in the center of the chest (green).
5. Throat chakra is located at the throat (blue).

6. Third Eye chakra is located between the eyebrows (indigo).
7. Crown chakra is located at the top of the head (purple).

Soon you will begin to notice a shift in the clothes and makeup colors you choose that will help you look and feel your best and further support your fullest and most colorful life.

CHAPTER 25

Music

The music of the soul can be heard through profound silence. What I mean by this is that when we are accustomed to and comfortable with the silence of our souls through meditation, the most beautiful harmony can then be created in our lives. And I don't just mean that if you are a musician and start a daily meditation ritual you will begin to produce chart-topping tunes. I mean that by allowing the silence to sing in our lives we will notice a greater rhythm flowing from within ourselves outwardly into a more balanced lifestyle.

On the other hand, many people find that when they do want to meditate it's virtually impossible to quiet the mind in silence; and then meditation becomes a chore. Believe it or not, just as we have colors that surround our bodies in auras, our auric field also emanates sound vibration. You're asking, "What does she mean by this? I can't hear music emanating from my partner next to me! Is she crazy?"

The energetic frequency that runs through us is created from our connection to source, and it carries a sound that on this earthly dimension isn't obvious to the human ear, but is to spirit and Mother Earth. Let's say, for example, that it is in your life's purpose and calling to be a musician. I knew someone whose life calling was most definitely to create music. He used to tell me he could hear it all the time in his mind, starting from when he was a young child. He was always downloading music from his soul and into the guitar and microphone. Because he was clearly living aligned with his soul's purpose, the natural creative flow was effortless, and being aligned through music came more easily for him than most.

However, let's say that it isn't your life's calling to be a rock star, but you love to listen to music. I mean, who doesn't really? How closely aligned we are with our soul's path will then determine what type of music we are attracted to. A common question when we meet someone new is often, "so what kind of music do you like?" I've always found that to be a difficult question to answer because I really do love all different kinds of music! One morning while writing I can be listening to New Age, and in the afternoon be popping it up with a Top 40 tune. If you are only attracted to one type of music, then chances are you are out of alignment with your source. Music is an energy that emanates from our souls, and the music we are attracted to can either nourish or deplete us on a soul level.

When I was in 7th grade I decided for my year-end science project that I would prove that the common houseplant could hear and respond to music! There were plenty of kids who came in with their parent-built volcanoes and pretend chemistry labs, but I sauntered in with my two plants and a boom box. For two weeks prior to my presentation, I'd set up two identical houseplants in the same spot in my windowsill for the same amount of time every other day. On the first day Plant One got to hear classical music, and on the second day Plant Two got to listen to hard rock! I did this for two weeks, and gave exactly the same amount of water to both plants and they were both exposed to the same amount of sunlight and my nurturing voice. I was only 12 years old, and for some reason I just knew that these plants were tuned into their environment. They were alive, pulsating at a frequency that I recognized, but nobody else seemed to.

The results of my experiment were as follows. Plant One with the classical music grew twice as large as Plant Two, which was exposed to hard rock and roll for two straight weeks. My teacher gave me a "C" and said that my experiment wasn't science at all, and that he didn't understand what I was talking about! I felt bad and humiliated, but I still knew inside that I was on to something and that it was my teacher who needed some enlightening!

Now, as an adult, I look back on that time and unbeknownst to me as a child, I subconsciously knew, even without any spiritual gurus or special knowledge whatsoever around me, that there was more to this life than what we can just perceive with our five senses. Because plants and minerals are expressions of source and Mother Earth that are completely free of human complications, it's no wonder that Plant One grew twice as much while listening to the quiet sounds of classical music than Plant Two. I'm not saying if you listen to rock and roll that you will become one with Satan! No, not at all, but if hard rock is all that you listen to for extended periods of time, it will deplete your energetic vibration; and so the need to get quiet every now and again would do you a world of good!

My point in telling you this story is to explain that music is essential to the world's evolution and peace. Every single musician, composer, and singer on this Earth is here as part of a collective agreement to help sustain Earth's musical vibration. When living in our individual existence we can consciously tune into our subconscious sound through meditation. On a collective level, we subconsciously influence musicians, composers, and singers to create certain types of music. So when we are in closer alignment with ourselves, we then have an effect on the music that permeates the time we live in.

It may sound complicated, but how many times have you heard someone refer to the music of a certain era, like the '60's '70's, and '80's? Music that is produced is subconsciously and energetically connected to the collective human consciousness of that time, and the people creating it are vehicles for that vibration.

Music is a tool that can promote healing on all levels by emanating joy, love, and even pain from within as all are necessary when purifying the soul of toxic, ego-based emotions. If it's music you need to help start off your meditation practice, or if you desire to continue to use it as way to further relax, then by all means do; and remember, the quieter the music, the louder your voice, creativity, and soul's purpose will become.

Because music changes and evolves right along with the development of human consciousness or lack thereof, it's up to you to create your own musical solstice from within. If the whole world were to do this, we might have the next Beatles revolution.

CHAPTER 26

Narcissism

Advanced by an endless stream of social of media, narcissism is a predominant theme in today's society. Social media dominates today's youth, fueling an unrealistic need to be liked. The level of attention and adornment required to fulfill one's neediness comes with an invincible price. YouTube, Facebook, and Instagram, for example, are 24/7 outlets for anyone to post and interact in a digital exchange that didn't exist 20 years ago. Narcissism, of course, existed 20 years ago, but back then it was only obvious in those with distinct personality traits.

The explosion of technology has brought forth a set of tools that cater to millions of egos, propelling today's youth into a dangerous direction—that of detachment from humanity and compassion, while setting unrealistic expectations and self-entitlement that may do more harm than good.

A girl posts a picture of herself and gets 122 "Likes," accompanied by hearts and lips in one day! But yesterday she got 153 Likes on a selfie that she posted! This sends her into a tailspin of self-deprecating thoughts and prompts her to head straight to her closet to doll herself up for yet another selfie because she needs to get the approval of those whose Likes she'd lost the day before. A scattered and distorted sense of self has been further warped by the influence of her ego, her Facebook friends, and a bunch of strangers.

When I was a teenager there were only monthly magazines to see fashion and beauty trends. Admittedly, the looks of the beautiful models influenced me on some level. I would spend hours after school copying the hair and makeup I saw on the models instead of doing my homework, and then would proudly present myself at the supper table! While I wanted to look like those models, I loved the art of the hair and makeup too!

Social media wasn't an available outlet for sharing my looks and creations. Not having that channel, which could potentially swell my ego, as well as my parents' concern for my homework not being being done, plus my sisters' condescension, my ego was kept realistically contained.

Looking at gorgeous models in magazines and watching beautiful movie stars can most certainly have an effect on a girl's self-esteem. In today's society, social media has such a powerful grip on people's insecurities that it has become an all-encompassing form of output and a fragmented outlet for uninteresting expression. Had I grown up in the age of selfies, no doubt I would have fallen into the social media ego trap of overly exploded self-adornment! But because there was only a monthly magazine to provide an influence on my external expressions, I had time to focus on more important things like my friends, school, boys, and sports!

So my point is this—a real sense of your own uniqueness will become completely false if you spend every day posting and waiting for virtual approval and acceptance. To be truly transparent and fully content with yourself you have to let go of the need for external approval and wander courageously into the realm of the unknown that waits within you. Begin by putting away your phone and computer once a week. And then extend it to an entire weekend!

Good old-fashioned reading from a book has been scientifically proven to send uplifting chemical neurons through the brainwaves, initiating a chain of positive thoughts and feelings throughout the body. Get off texting and actually talk to your friends the old-fashioned way! And most importantly, acknowledge that you are a beautiful, sentient being whose beauty can never be judged by pure love; it can only be judged by the ego.

CHAPTER 27

Ancient Egyptian Beauty Rituals

Ancient Egypt was one of the first societies on Earth that is remembered for rendering a unique assortment of beautiful artifacts, rituals, and fashion. Many of the aromas that Egyptians used like, myrrh, jasmine, and neroli, are still used today to enhance modern fragrances.

Fascinating beauty rituals and traditions were actualized in Egyptians' daily routines. Beauty was coveted and its practices were very different from today's beauty trends. Theirs was a society that embraced spiritual practices and rituals as a means to honor the beauty that they were trying to achieve. A profound belief in gods and goddesses enriched their practices of adornment and greatly influenced the art, fashion, and beauty of their time. It's believed that the Ancient Egyptians' traditions around beauty allowed for ease and comfort in their communion with both the gods and their spiritual selves.

A great lady of ancient Egypt could have had more than a dozen servants and ladies in waiting to help her practice her daily beauty rituals. Because beauty rituals were intimately connected to spiritual practices, the ancients understood the spiritual beliefs and practices to be an interactive pathway between inner and outer beauty. In fact, without the spiritual practices and assistance from gods and goddesses, they believed they would die.

An ancient Egyptian beauty would have placed great importance on her daily beauty rituals. Beginning with prayer, silence, burning of incense, and mixing of oils and paints, she would have taken time to nurture her inner self, thus revealing her authentic beauty.

Are these ancient traditions, practices, and beliefs really so farfetched that today's woman couldn't adapt some of these artistic rituals to her own daily life? It's true that unless you are Queen Elizabeth or wealthy Saudi princess, modern women around the world do not require ladies in waiting and servants. However, adopting the idea of peacefully connecting your daily beauty routine with a spiritual act is plausible, and can be beneficial to the upliftment of consciousness and external beauty.

Upon awakening in the morning an Egyptian woman would have headed straight into her temple to pray to the gods and receive blessings for a new day, as it was believed that each day was a new beginning of life and breath. Then she would have proceeded with the delicate, honoring process of beautifying her surroundings with scent and adorning herself respectfully with the makeup, jewelry and fashions that she believed best reflected the goddess within her. Can you imagine adding a spiritual practice into your own morning routine to honor your inner goddess?

When I awake each day, I do so 45 minutes before anyone else does, except for my cat of course! I meditate and pray every morning. Then I pour myself some coffee and listen to quiet music, and start to clean myself up. I guard this time as the most important of my day, as it allows me to center my inner self, my intuition, and it gives me time to appreciate myself and my looks as I put my mascara on. So, is my morning routine really all that different from the goddesses of Ancient Egypt? No it isn't.

Investing time in something greater than what only your ego can comprehend assists you and the universe in creating a more peaceful and beautiful existence. Take your time, slow down, and begin to breathe. Let the silence of a beautiful and tranquil morning guide you to your inner, most beautiful self for there she waits to be adorned with love and care.

CHAPTER 28

Balance

Balance in our lives comes and goes much like the money in my bank account when I was a struggling artist! Because money, like love, health, and happiness, is just another form of energetic frequency, now when I see my flow being slowed down, I'll ask myself, "Where am I off balance in my life?" Managing a family and career, and focusing on your life's purpose can throw a whole lot of teeter-totter into the balance and flow of life. Therefore, creating stability in your spirit is the key to expressing and fulfilling a healthful and balanced life.

You can achieve a comfortable level of balance in your life if you focus on being organized and cognizant of over-scheduling, but if you continue to neglect yourself and your source over an extended period of time, then the balance you so efficiently created will eventually fall out of order. For some, it may come up in health issues; for others, frequent breakups; some may be control freaks; and for some it may show up as a lack of flow in finances.

It's not easy tapping into the source of your imbalance either! For me, I came to the conclusion that one of my imbalances was in the area of receiving, and from time to time that would manifest as a lack of money. When you are constantly giving to others and taking care of everyone else's needs, remembering to stay open to receiving may not be so easily done in your daily life. Giving, however, must have a balance, and that is where receiving comes in!

Where is your unbalance revealing itself? The first thing, situation, or person that comes to your mind is most likely what is manifesting as your imbalance. How do we fix these chronic episodes and lack of balance in our lives?

Once you have reached a level in your meditation practice where you can deeply connect to your source, the time when you almost feel as if you would fall asleep is the moment when you can mentally ask, "What is the source of my imbalance?" If the answer doesn't come immediately, it will present itself in a day or two through an example or sign of some sort.

When you are in tune with your practice you then elevate your energetic frequency enough for the universe to respond to the uncluttered vibration of love pouring out of your soul; and when this occurs your episodes of imbalance will diminish! They will not disappear completely because we are housed in a human body with a human mind. But we will always be presented with opportunities to learn and grow and fix the imbalances when they come up. You will become more aware and less stressed out when things are tipping the scale in the wrong direction. Your episodes of imbalance won't last as long and will not be as painful.

Your soul is abundant and infinite, balanced by the power of omniscient light. It shines through you like a glittering star on a dark night, brightening the world ahead of you. All you have to do is awaken to it, and the alignment will take its place firmly within your heart, reminding you daily of the awesome, beautiful power that you are made of.

CHAPTER 29

Animal Spirit

Every animal on Earth, no matter what type, is here as part of a collective giving to humanity and Mother Earth, bridging and balancing the energies between heaven and Earth. Have you ever noticed that children are innocently drawn to bunny rabbits, puppies, kittens, and seemingly all other animals they become acquainted with? We use stuffed animals to soothe our kids to sleep, and depend on these cute, fluffy toys to calm their souls and welcome sweet dreams.

But have you ever thought deeply about the unequivocal role that animals play in our lives, beauty, and consciousness? If you have not known the love of a loyal pet, then your soul has not yet been blessed with a kiss of universal love, for it is in animals that the uncluttered, pure vibration of love can easily display itself.

Unfortunately there are still big corporations who use and exploit animals for unnecessary research, all for more global human consumption and greed. Believing that animals are of a lesser consciousness than ourselves and not as important as we are makes it easier for humans to look the other way and ignore the plight that many animals on the planet still face. Awareness is growing in the scientific community, and slowly there seems to be some understanding that animals are sentient beings and that using and exploiting them for our profit is wrong.

Allow yourself to remain open for just a moment to observe or listen to the spiritual quality of animals and how they influence the collective consciousness. It may surprise and uplift your spirit, even for just that moment. My cat, for instance, is an expression of uncomplicated love! When I hold her, the vibration of complete calm and peace exudes from her heart as she comforts my spirit and increases my joy.

Animals communicate in a different way than humans. Of course, we all know this. Being able to purely and solely listen to your intuition, to communicate from intuition, is a gift that many humans do not enjoy, but animals do! Just imagine being able to communicate through your intuition and soul awareness with people as easily as with your pet?

Let me give you an example of what I'm talking about. Once my cat suddenly became sick with a high fever and was very listless. I meditated for a long period of time with her in my arms before taking her to the vet. When I reached a place of complete release, I mentally asked her what was wrong and what she needed. She responded mentally, telling me she had developed some inflammation in her body that was due to a virus. She said she needed rest and an ice pack to cool her body, and that my love would help her the most. I started the ice therapy, and within a few hours she seemed a little better. However, my human mind got worried, and I began to distrust my communication with her, so I took her into the vet. After several tests, a sad night in the animal hospital, and $1,000 later, the doctor concluded that he was baffled because everything was normal according to the science of things. He wanted to keep her in the hospital because of the fever, but I refused. I knew at that moment that my original contact with her was indeed correct. Two days later she was hopping and running around, and back to her old, loveable self!

My point in telling you this story is this. If we all were able to elevate our consciousness on a collective level, our relationship to animals would universally change. Slaughterhouses would cease to exist and the overproduction of meat for human consumption would stop.

It's true that our ancestors ate meat, but much less frequently than modern day humans. A lovely, young girl once told me a story that took place in her small village in South America. I can't remember the country, but her story stuck with me. She explained that where she came from, they ate goat meat. There, goats were raised gently and naturally, or what we'd consider "organic," and with love. When it was time to sacrifice the goat for food, they performed a spiritual ceremony, thanking the goat and the Earth for its bounty. They believed that the goats knew on a soul level why they were there and, ultimately, their meat was needed to help nourish humans. What about the animals in slaughterhouses being battered and abused? They exist because of humanity's free will— free will to do with the animals what we choose to do, operating from ignorance and greed.

If we all began to nurture our own souls on a daily basis, eventually, but maybe not in my lifetime, humans would on a collective level begin to honor the animals much like in that South American village, and begin to see all animals as sacred, energetic beings. As long as there are slaughterhouses, there will be wars on Earth and innocent humans will die! That's because it is part of the energetic exchange that humans must face for the collective ignorance and abuse of the great animal spirit that is profoundly needed for sustainable peace and advancement of consciousness.

For centuries, Native Americans have honored animals and their spirits in animal totems. They believe that each animal is represented as a totem and that each human has a certain totem, or several, at various times in their lives, present and available for their spiritual nourishment and guidance. In your meditation practices, you can call upon the spirit of any animal to assist you in any area of your life. For example, you can call upon the spirit of lion to come forth in your meditation, which spiritually represents strength, courage, determination, and fierce beauty.

Let's say there is a new job you really want more than anything. Call upon lion energy to assist you with your confidence and unleash your own inner lion or lioness. And remember, the next time you cast out the thought of an animal as not being conscious, it is really you who is detached from your own higher consciousness. Donate your time at an animal shelter once a week, become a foster volunteer, or adopt a pet! Spending more time with animals reduces stress and promotes feelings of joy and peace, and it will help you spiritually align with the uncluttered part of your spirit that needs nourishment and attention.

CHAPTER 30

Jewelry

When Marilyn Monroe sang the famous tune "Diamonds are a girl's best friend," she wasn't kidding around! Jewels of all kinds, colors, shapes, and sizes have been part of our fashion expression since the Ancient Egyptian era as I mentioned before. Did you know that jewelry, and particularly precious gems like diamonds and amethysts, carry and absorb actual energy?

Recently, I met a woman who owns a beautiful jewelry shop in New York City. I noticed that her shop didn't have any healing crystals, like topaz or quartz, in any of the jewelry cases. I mentioned that if she put these in with the other jewelry, she might sell more and have better interactions with customers. She had no idea that jewelry carries, conducts, and absorbs energy.

Because stones and gems come from the earth, they inherit magnetized energy from Earth's core crystal, which lies at the very center of our planet. It ignites the crystals and gems much like the sun helps vegetation to grow. So when we wear a piece of jewelry that is made of raw material from the earth, we transport that energy with us, and even absorb it into our own auras and physical bodies.

That's why when choosing a piece of jewelry it behooves us to learn where it came from and how it was produced.

If you are wearing diamonds, for example, you may want to know if they were excavated from a poor country by exploited and abused child slave labor. Because the gems will have absorbed a level of negative and malignant energy, it will then begin transmuting itself into your being and your life as you wear it. The energy transmutation won't be obvious to most, but if you wear a piece of jewelry on your body that hasn't been cleared of negative vibrations, over a long period of time physical malaise can appear, perhaps, in the form of migraine headaches, ulcers, or other unexplainable physical and emotional ailments.

Or, let's say that your fiancé innocently finds a beautiful vintage aquamarine engagement ring. And let's say that ring came from a woman who was physically abused for her entire marriage. The ring has absorbed that energy, and now you and your fiancé have inherited some negative vibes! It won't cause you to get divorced, but unbeknownst to you, it can insidiously infuse its negative vibration into your relationship.

On the other hand, if you are wearing a piece of jewelry that has been excavated with integrity and cleansed energetically, then the crystals, stones, and gems can infuse you with a pure, energetic beauty and uplifting vibration that assists in aligning your mind, body, and soul with the all-encompassing power of source and Mother Earth.

One of the easiest ways to clear your jewelry of any negative vibrations is through an intention to clear and prayer, and by leaving your precious gems in a combination of moonlight and sunlight over a 24-hour period.

When choosing jewelry to buy, acknowledge that the gems are alive too, and let them call to you through your intuition. When you do that, rest assured that there is a purpose your soul wishes to fulfill in becoming aligned with certain gems and colors. Remember they come from the earth and have a purpose similar to the animals in our lives. They are not called precious stones and gems just because they may be expensive; it's more because they can have such a powerful influence on our wellbeing and, ultimately, our beauty!

CHAPTER 31

Patience

Patience used to be one of my least favorite words! Back in time when I was actively searching for love, for example, a well-known psychic told me that I had to be patient for my husband to come into my life, that I needed to focus more on my own self-development, and that the timing wasn't here yet for me to be married with a family. I needed to become more patient—ah!

Patience is a virtue, so they say, but the truth is that after all my years of living in New York, it's something I have had to constantly cultivate within myself. Patience isn't convenient in a modern world, and is intensified in a fast-paced megacity. Even waiting for the Six train for more than three minutes can literally emotionally derail even the most spiritually evolved of New Yorkers! So what to do?

When you want something to happen in your life, you have to set the intention with the utmost of clarity and conviction that nothing can or will get in the way of what you wish to manifest into your life; and you have to be willing to be patient. Because the universe has a thing called "divine timing," no matter how powerful your conviction is you cannot speed up the road map of your life's purpose. You see, before you came into this life you made a soul contract and map of how your life could look—assuming, of course, that you would become conscious and in tune with your soul enough that you'd remember your chosen path.

When we fall off our path and become detached from our source, we are no longer directly aligned with the life map that we created. And that is when we become anxious, nervous, and stressed about how things are currently working in our lives. We might try and pretend to be patient because we've heard that's what we're supposed to do when things aren't happening quickly enough to our liking. Impatience, nevertheless, is deeply embedded in the consciousness of most; in other words, it's a typical human reaction, especially in a hurried world. Ironically, for most of us, arriving at that calm, blissful state of patience takes practice.

You can't rush life. You have to be patient and allow life to lead you onto your soul's divine path, the one that's been ordained for you. By practicing the art of being patient—which I believe it truly is—we welcome a more subconscious quiet into our energetic vibration, which in turn leads us to our soul's divine path and the set of circumstances that will deliver us to our true sense of self, and, ultimately, to our joy.

How do we practice the art of being patient? By now you will have guessed that the answer is, yes, meditation. Meditation is the most powerful tool we have to help us grow more patient. By attuning to the silence within on a daily basis we can more easily access our life's blueprint, and then the art of patience becomes our ally, not our enemy! We evolve enough to know and accept that certain things that we desire to occur in our life will indeed occur when the timing is right and not before. When we are patient that which we desire flows to us with grace through the ether of the cosmos because it has been already written by your soul for your greatest learning and upliftment.

CHAPTER 32

Listening

The gift of hearing is one of God's most glorious gifts! Listening to favorite music, our kids laughing, the birds chirping, and even the silence are all part of a unified center of being that inputs into our cells an opportunity to download joy into our daily lives through listening. But how many people are actually accomplished in the art of listening? Practically everyone wants their point of view to be heard and accepted, and many literally do not stop talking until they can either get the other party to accept their view, or they just annoy everyone around them, disrupting relationships and even their own personal balance. OK so listen up, everyone, I have a news flash!

You cannot incorporate divine information into your cellular being unless you have reached a point in your meditation practice that will allow you to process sound of any kind into your mind, body, and soul structure. What do I mean by this? When you have unlocked your higher self through the practice of meditation you will recognize it in the way you live your own life. Things, people, and activities will no longer resonate with your happiness like they once did, and you will notice that being silent or practicing silence will become your new norm. Listening then becomes automatic, as it is an inherent ability designed to support your continued evolvement in this lifetime.

People who talk too much and are unwilling to listen will become an obvious indicator for you to either subconsciously let go, or you will feel inclined to guide or teach them. People who talk too much use their power of speech to deflect the enormous disparity between their ego and their true selves. It is a comfort zone that places the ego where it loves to thrive, where ignorance and arrogance are on the forefront of one's existence. They may say during an argument that they hear you, but their actions will prove otherwise because they are not vibrationally connected to their true selves.

On the other hand, people who are good listeners are often great teachers, are more intuitive, not selfish and self-centered, do not participate in gossip, enjoy giving, and often live quite simplistically. Learning to listen to yourself is the first step to becoming a great listener. Your inner voice is the most powerful of all; yet it is quiet and vibrates outwardly through your core, manifesting itself through your heart center in the form of feelings and emotions. Becoming aligned with this valuable tool is often more important than hearing something with your physical ears because it keeps you attuned to the truth flowing within you and others around you.

By developing your sixth sense through meditation, the art of listening becomes second-nature and a great friend. Start by imagining during your meditation a golden light flowing in and out of your ears. Breathe the light in and out, unblocking the heavy weight of the ego. Then bring the light down through your heart center, continuing to breathe in and out slowly and consciously. Affirm this mantra during your meditation for 10 minutes: "I hear only love."

At the end of 10 minutes, gently release the mantra. You may find that after first practicing this meditation that you might not feel much like talking that day. This means you are on your way to becoming powerfully aware of the beauty of quietly listening. Your attunement will change, and you'll begin to hear things that you never did before.

CHAPTER 33

Spiritually Strong

What does it mean to be spiritually strong? Someone I recently encountered who had just returned from Burning Man said to me that anyone seeking enlightenment couldn't achieve it without a trip to this unifying clique of soul-seekers searching for an intense release and a sense of pure spiritual bliss. The spiritual-seekers have the correct intention, but is the direction of their intention actually correct?

I am certain that I am spiritually strong! Why I am a confident in saying this? It's not because I vacation once a year at Burning Man or have had the privilege of visiting Machu Picchu! It is because I have devoted more than two decades now to my meditation practice. Making this a priority in my life has strengthened me in many ways.

When you are spiritually strong you are able to face life's challenges head on with understanding, compassion, and a fierce knowing that all will be well. Meditation has made me more intuitive, more patient, more joyful, more creative, and it has strengthened my ability to love beyond anything I ever could have imagined for myself. It has taught me that humility is one of the greatest gifts we can ascertain, and that giving is an essential part of our existence on Earth. Going within everyday has given me the strength and enlightenment that I never thought possible before I started on this journey.

Maybe a trip to Burning Man would be fun and heighten my sense of self, but to believe that a trip to a famous "spiritual" place on Earth will awaken you to your higher self is a mistake. Seeking spiritual strength takes a serious, gentle, and loving commitment to yourself much like when you embark upon the commitment of marriage.

When you are spiritually strong, you feel more beautiful! Because you identify your true beauty with the beating of your heart and your love and compassion first, your outward appearance becomes the second thing you think about. The beauty that pulsates at a frequency beyond the outer reflection you see in the mirror is, in fact, the cure for any insecurity, pain, or disillusionment you may feel about the way you look.

Focusing on your strengths on a daily basis instead of your weaknesses is an easy way to deflect unhappy or less than desirable thoughts about yourself. Focus on what is flowing in your life, what is going right, instead of only seeing what is going wrong. The same goes for your looks! Instead of focusing on what you don't like about yourself, begin by focusing on what you do like.

For example, let's say that you have small lips and you obsess about wanting bigger lips. You get lip injections to try and achieve a fuller lip, as you're convinced it will make you feel better. After you get your injections, it does make you feel better! Or, at least it makes your ego feel better. But your higher self doesn't give a hoot about having bigger lips. Your source loves you just the way you are, and actually wants you to shift your negative focus on your lips to your big, beautifully shaped eyes instead! This shift in positive, loving vibrations you give yourself brings you closer to the true and beautiful you.

Spiritual strength comes from you and only you, and your belief in yourself, your love of yourself, and your compassion for yourself! Know that it is something you can always count on— as long as you pay attention to it every day and never let go.

CHAPTER 34

State of Mind

It's never too early to start your spiritual practice! My daughter has become quite familiar with mine, and now she will voluntarily sit with me from time to time and meditate with me. Even just a few moments of sitting in the stillness can open the channel for your soul to sing sweetly to your heart and mind. The earlier in life you can become acquainted with your higher self the better, for then the life path becomes more peaceful and power of the ego is diminished.

It's never too late to start either, for to spend your entire life not knowing why you are here is like a ship that never had sails! Believing what the ego wants us to achieve, which is to absorb as much material wealth as we can and to look as young as we can for as long as we can, is a massive misconception and misuse of the intelligence of source.

We are here to embrace our angelic beauty that illuminates from within and shines outwardly, paving the way and caressing other souls to amplify their potentiality into actuality. Actualizing the pure potential to thrive, succeed, give, and love is the way to access the unlimited source of wealth and beauty of the spirit. It is not a mathematical equation or a mysterious quantum physics dispute.

Feeling the beauty you are made of is simple; yet the power of the ego can easily trick you into a false understanding of the beauty of your true source and the false beauty of the ego. The false beauty of the ego represents an inevitable distraction and constant reminder for even the most spiritually evolved that the evolution of your soul depends greatly on your ability to recognize those energies that do not align with your source, which is your true beauty.

Money isn't needed to buy more beauty. Real beauty is in loving acts of kindness, in service to others, in the joy you feel when you've made someone laugh! Our external beauty is something that we have been genetically predisposed to and something we have chosen on a soul level. If you are not happy with the way you look or are unaligned with your higher self, you will feel the constant need to change, alter, or express your external beauty in a way that triggers discomfort and ongoing dissatisfaction. You will not stop until you allow your source to come knocking loudly from within in such a way that it knocks you right out of your mind and into your capacity to understand.

Being balanced from within through the consistent practice of meditation will allow the state of mind to become more peaceful and receptive to the energy that you are made of, and thus will create a happier, more beautiful and peaceful existence. Mastering Beauty is a state of balanced mind, body, and spirit! Mastering your true beauty from within is a complete and peaceful state of being that allows your source to flourish like baby blossoms of spring. It is an accomplished sense of self that exemplifies humility, grace, generosity, and above all, allows love to reside in the one and only beautiful you!

The Ultimate Beauty

The ultimate beauty, the quintessential space between your inner self and your outer shell is awaiting your attention right now!

Go there and be.
Just be
Still.
Love and honor yourself.
Be still in the silence.
Allow it to envelop you from deep within and penetrate and release the fear and unwanted.
You are the ultimate beauty.
It is you.
In you,
Of you,
Around you,
Surrounding you,
Awaiting you.
Beneath the surface of aggravated disguise
Is the true beauty you are made of:
The power

The strength
The love.
Own it.
Embrace it.
The divine love
In you.
Begin by going in
And let the silence resonate for just a moment and let your source whisper to you gently.
Then await the roar! Because once it is unleashed you will never dare to compare yourself again to anyone or anything!
You are the Master of your own beauty!

CHAPTER 36

Relaxation

Do you ever feel guilty when you relax? Relaxing our minds and bodies is an essential need for our inner and outer wellbeing and health! Regular time away from technology, work, and people is requisite for living a healthful and balanced life. This is why meditation is such a radically effective way to relax. Meditation not only assists you in tuning in to your source and aligns you with your life's path, but it also supports your physical mind and body.

Prayer is also important in helping you to relax, but praying without first elevating your vibration from within is not as powerful a call to source as when you are consciously aligned. If there were a time on Earth when everyone collectively meditated at the same time, peace rather than war, famine, and corruption, would become more prevalent in all societies.

After you meditate you should, without shame or guilt, incorporate other relaxing activities into your life that bring you a feeling of joy and gratitude. Whether it's a trip to a yoga class or the nail salon, a bit of self-love and care should be a part of your regular schedule. I used to have an agent many years ago who would take a 20-minute nap on the floor every day in his office. He'd tell me that to fall asleep quickly he would envision a beautiful sunset descending upon a landscape of cascading mountains. He said that it refreshed and relaxed him in the middle of the day when fatigue and stress would often creep in.

You may be thinking, "I can't possibly take a nap in the middle of the day!" But science shows that resting when your body and mind need it can, in fact, reduce the signs of aging, both physically and mentally. The truth is the more you place importance on regular relaxation, the more productive and creative in your life you will become. Burnout promotes inauthentic, haphazard results, while a relaxed state of mind and body lifts your work to its highest potential.

This same principle can be used when thinking about your relationships. Particularly for mothers, this can be a tricky or daunting thought! Relaxation is actually a terrifying word for some! If you don't find some regular time to relax, you can't function as your authentic self, and therefore your relationships with your kids, friends, and partners will not flow as authentically as they should. Therefore, take time to relax every day and truly enjoy those moments that you are dedicating to yourself. You matter! Your life matters! Your health matters! You are a powerful soul that can only manifest itself in a relaxed environment and that environment is you!

CHAPTER 37

The Princess Beauty

The idea of growing up to become a princess is one that many little girls desire at one point or another in their young lives. It's an ideology presented to humankind on a commercial level that implicates the feminine as weak or less serious. When we think of a princess, we tend to connect to the Disney kind of princess, a fairytale kind of character that enjoys a life of royalty, regal settings, beautiful things, and, of course, the perfect prince. What's dangerous about this message to girls is that it's introduced at a young age when it has the potential to deeply engrave itself within the ego where it may settle for long periods of time, lasting years, or perhaps even a lifetime, if not purposely and spiritually relinquished.

There are plenty of modern day, so-called princesses acting out on television, in reality shows, and through social media. We see tantrums, elevated narcissism, excessive spending, too much makeup, and surgically enhanced looks. These females are a prime example of what can happen when too much Princess Dom has penetrated the ego, and the human shell becomes a vehicle of harsh and extreme imbalances.

When a girl believes from a young age that she can have whatever she desires in life without ever hearing the word "no," she is set up for a life of self-entitlement that can and will lead to disappointment and failure in certain areas, depending on the karmic path. We all want to feel special, and the idea of "princess" exemplifies this, but what gets lost in translation is that often the world's most famous princesses have been, or are, lost in the actual translation of the title they've been given.

What do I mean by this? Let's take Her Royal Highness the late Princess Diana. She was probably the most famous princess in history. Women the world over looked to her as an example and for hope for their own lives on multiple levels of existence. She came forth as Princess Diana in her lifetime as part of a karmic agreement to assist in uplifting the consciousness of humankind. She brought a new dimension to the crown, a warm and human element, demonstrating that being a princess was more an expression of a divine mission rather than a life of pageantry and entitlement. We were introduced to a woman with real feelings and heart, a woman who was vulnerable and unsure, a woman who desired what many women do: a family life filled with love and happiness, children who grow to become good and honest people and do good things for others, and a purposeful life in which a woman can feel good about herself and her accomplishments.

Being a "princess" is a term that can actually victimize females into believing that their power lies solely in their physical beauty, and not in their mission and purpose in life. What's important to remember is that loving who you are and reminding yourself every day is far more important than a title, or acting falsely and pretending to be a reality show princess. For all intents and purposes, Princess Diana has become an icon of hope, peace, and beauty. So the next time your little girl watches a Disney movie, remind her afterwards that there once lived a real princess named Diana who was kind, generous, funny and lived a short life with an intense spiritual mission to uplift consciousness and bring more awareness and acceptance to humankind.

The true beauty of a princess, of every girl, unfolds when she is following her soul's path toward enlightenment. Know that each and every one of you can create your own legacy and "princess beauty" through loving acts of kindness.

CHAPTER 38

The Magical Beauty

Humans are embodied with an exquisite energy that moves through them and is exchanged at an alternate frequency that isn't typically visible to or felt by everyone. Nevertheless, each person has the capability to transform his or her perception of self from strictly physical to an energetic being as well. There are individuals on the planet who are able to see their own auras and those of others. They are attuned to an elevated frequency, which enables them to also communicate with energies outside their own physical body and mind.

Just imagine a world where when you awoke every morning and looked in the mirror, instead of seeing what a physical mess you are in, you would examine the richness and colors of your own energy field—your own truest beauty! The source of your beauty is a euphoric field of energy that encases you. You can learn to see it, as well as access it through meditation.

The glow of your field of source can also be seen surrounding the iris of your physical eye by simply gazing into the eye without judgment and fear. To begin to actually see the energy you are made of, you must first begin your meditation practice. By now I have clearly ingrained this into your consciousness, or at least I hope so! Because without elevating your connection to your higher self you cannot truly enjoy the benefits of living a purposeful, soul-filled life and accomplish the all-important mastery of beauty from deep within.

After you have developed a daily, nonnegotiable meditation ritual for a period of time, you'll have altered your vibration from within enough to be able to recognize a change occurring within you. To do this, instead of quickly dismissing yourself as a mess in the morning and jumping straight to the makeup for help, gently, yet steadily gaze at your third eye center between your eyebrows as you stand upright and not too close to the mirror. Without crossing your eyes, relax your gaze and start to notice the reflective brilliant color of your source completely surrounding your body.

Once you have accomplished this magnificent step, you'll be drawn to examining your aura each morning rather than your physical faults. One morning your reflection may contain pink, and the next yellow, and so on. This could be the new measurement of how beautiful you feel in the morning! The stronger your pulsation of color, the more beauty you emanate. You are a magical beauty, truly capable of altering your own reality without the use of mind-altering drugs or artificial substances because your source is more powerful than any outside tool you believe will help you.

The magic is in you, right there and ready for you to wield however you desire. All it takes is a daily dedication to care and enrich your spirit as much as you would your skin and hair. Follow this mantra to assist in opening the channel to your deepest you: "In me resides the magic of love and true beauty!"

CHAPTER 39

Transgender Beauty

Defining beauty from a female and male perspective is how we most readily represent our souls on the human level of existence. But consider for just a moment that all souls are, in fact, genderless. Souls can choose to represent themselves as female, male, animal, or even as the ocean.

On a soul level humans can reincarnate multiple times as both male and female. This is to help the soul evolve spiritually, and to balance the kinetic exchange of energies that exist in the microcosm of cells that comprise a soul. So when we see a man in the public eye who's been famous for representing a strong masculine presence for an extended period of time, who then chooses to change his gender to female, it can be difficult and uncomfortable to mentally and emotionally comprehend. But consider the soul's journey of transcending time, physical reality, and evolution as the first and foremost important factor in choice and free will.

Encompassing both female and male energies in one physical body is challenging for even the most spiritually evolved human, yet it is a state of existence that truly embodies the fully evolved soul—a place where the embodiment is comfortable and at peace with its existence no matter what physical gender it's born into. In the case of a soul that feels it is in the wrong body, this is a situation that the individual soul creates to accelerate the embodiment of male and female attachment, to karmically attune with and surrender to the spiritual path and higher self, and to karmically release all negative exchanges from past lives that only the soul remembers and the human mind does not.

It's not a case of being trapped in the wrong body, even though those experiencing that state might disagree. It is, simply put, a state of existence chosen by the soul in this lifetime to master the beauty of the soul and express its power and will to transmute all physical boundaries imposed by society and culture. The beauty presents itself into two alternative sexes to engage humanity on a collective level to reach a point in evolution where what the culture defines as beautiful no longer exists. It further promotes tolerance and acceptance among those who are in great need of an open-ended existence.

The transgender human is, spiritually speaking, a transient being expressing the desire to promote a complementary existence to the imbalance of the collective human ego, and to express oneself outside the generally accepted standards of beauty that humans are used to. Transgender souls are mastering their own unique beauty and realizing their power through their courage, faith, and conviction in their ability to live in and express their soul's truth and life path.

If you are a soul experiencing the transgender life path, then a daily meditation practice grounded in the intention of communing with your soul is highly recommended because of the extreme discomfort this life path can create. The ego wants you to fail in your mission to uplift consciousness, but the power of source, once turned on, can diminish the darkest of days.

Start by sitting in a comfortable, upright position, and breathe deeply in and out for several minutes. Focus solely on your breath. Ask your divine self to come through with these words: "I ask my

Golden Solar Angel to be with me now." Rest here, and continue breathing.

Imagine the most powerful, benevolent of golden angels hovering over your head. The angel that is your higher self is uncluttered, free of guilt, shame, and confusion. Allow the angel's golden light to flood through your entire body, starting from the top of your head, and flowing downward. Gently, deeply, breathe it all in. Ask your Golden Solar Angel to be with you everyday. Begin to see and feel a shift within yourself, and know how deeply you are loved and how important you are to humankind's evolution.

GUIDED MEDITATION
GETTING STARTED

To begin a successful meditation practice one must first decide why it is they want to embark upon this path. Meditation isn't something you do once in awhile; it is a constant, ever-flowing practice, much like a yoga practice. You begin with a set of realistic attitudes and goals towards your newfound desire to connect to your higher vibration. And then be willing to let go of controlling of a desired outcome. If you expect to become enlightened in just a few days, you are incorrect. But you will experience a lighter sense of relaxation in the very beginning. The real and more sustaining results come after some time and after considerable effort has been put into practice. Eventually the resistance to sitting will subside, and you will view your meditation practice as a way of existence that guides and assists you through the rest of your life path.

I recommend in the beginning to start your practice seated in a chair that will allow you to sit upright and will easily assist you in keeping your spine erect. You want to avoid sitting in a chair or couch that can swallow you into a lazy slouch. This will lead to a passive form of meditation, and you can easily fall asleep. If you are flexible, the ideal position for your meditation practice will be to sit on a meditation cushion with legs crossed underneath you. You do not have to be in full lotus position to receive the benefits of meditation.

Your bottom should be elevated slightly above your thighs and legs, as shown in the diagram. Your hands should be placed in a cupped position in your lap, and tucked in front of your naval. With your eyes closed begin to focus on your breath, feeling the breath flowing in and out of your nose.

We use our breath as the main focal point for our minds to allow the awakening of the molecular conjunction between our higher, universal mind and our human mind to vibrationally mesh into a spherical opening that allows for the two to coexist during meditation. In other words, to get out of the human mind and the demands of the ego, focusing on our breath assists us to tap into our higher self and mind, to set up a landing dock of sorts, for the human mind and ego to be placed so that our source can power through and awaken us to its strength and beauty.

Sit quietly.
Breathe in and out,
focusing on the breath flowing in and out,
over and over.
Breathe.

When your mind strays, notice the thought, then get immediately back to your breath. Start for 10 minutes each day for one week. Use this time to get acquainted with your breath and your posture. Be patient with yourself, and wait.

A successful meditation practice develops over time, and much like a diet or exercise program, results are not instantaneous. Nonetheless, taming the mind and ego is a process well worth the effort and the determination to succeed.

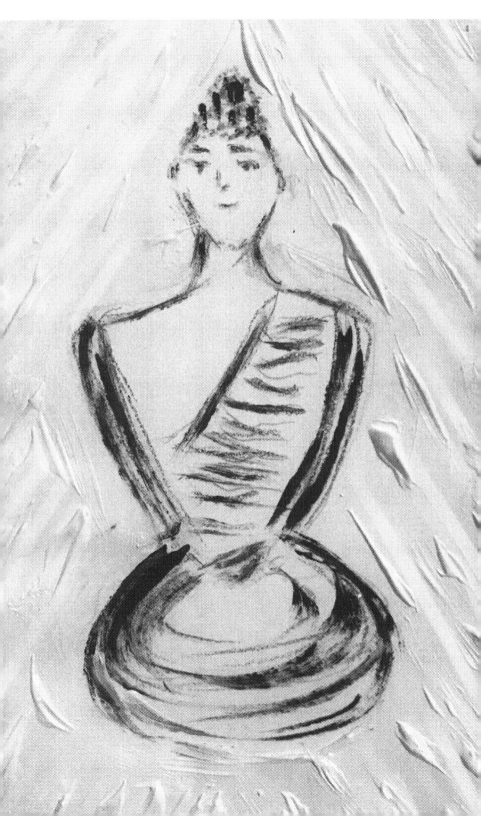

Meditation for Intuition

Sit comfortably in an upright position, and shake your hands three times.

Take three deep breaths in and out.

Close your eyes.

Imagine a beautiful, blue, magical doorway being presented to you.

Mentally walk through the door and feel a warm, majestic, blue light surround your body.

Begin to breath in this magnificent, blue light by envisioning it coming through the middle of the top of your eyebrows, the area called your "third eye."

Continue to focus the blue light in and out, and let the light shine from within your entire head outwards.

If your mind begins to wander, incorporate counting into the meditation.

Start from one and breathe in the blue light, and on two exhale. Continue to 10, and start back at one if you need to.

When you have finished, mentally walk back through the blue door and open your eyes.

After you have finished you should feel a tingling at the top of your head.

You have just activated and opened the channel for greater intuition into your life.

Your intuition is your open line of communication between your source and outside influences affecting your daily life and path.

Use this meditation technique once per week.

And begin to notice a greater rhythm of positive flow towards achieving your desires and manifesting them into reality.

Meditation for Manifestation

Begin seated in a comfortable position with your back in a straight, upright position and with your body facing north.

To proceed, close your eyes and stomp your feet one at a time, six times each, to release any stagnant energy in the legs.

Then forcefully clap your hands together six times to ignite the flow of energy and bliss through the body.

Take six deep breaths, inhaling deeply and exhaling forcefully.

Close your eyes, and imagine a beautiful circle of green light swirling in front of your chest as if a tornado is approaching.

Then slowly breathe in this green light and swirling energy.

Allow your body to deeply relax with the energy growing stronger within.

You should begin to feel the mind and body gently relaxing.

After your meditation, affirm six times that which you desire to manifest into your life.

For example:

"I intend to allow a positive flow of money into my life using my abilities and talents."

Continue to use this manifestation and affirmation meditation regularly to put your energetic intentions out into the universe.

Guided Visualization and Meditation
for Healing and Detoxifying

Sit with your back in an upright position.

Close your eyes.

Listen to the ocean in your mind; mentally hear the waves gently breaking on the shore of your consciousness.

Breathe in the fresh smell of the ocean air, and hear the seagulls

Sing sweetly.

Immerse yourself completely in the quiet, powerful calm of the healing and detoxifying energy of the ocean.

Breath deeply in and out.

Then begin mentally to walk into the ocean,

Slowly and calmly feeling the warmth and gentle touch of the water's grace.

Feel the sand wiggling freely beneath your feet.

Then when you feel relaxed and completely free of the heavy weight in your body,

Dive with great joy and courage into the depths of the ocean.

Feel the cool and refreshing touch of the sea salt water

Caressing your skin and replenishing your soul.

Swim.

Now gently bring your body onto its back and float upon the top of the water, allowing it to fully support you and your body.

Be here and breathe.

Feel the energy you are made of.

Allow the current to guide you and lead you deeper into your soul's awakening.

You are one with the ocean's force, its peace and its beauty.

Connect with this vibration whenever your energy is depleted.

As you come back to consciousness,

Thank the ocean for its bounty, and bless its energy. As you do, you will assist it in elevating its frequency along with yours.

Namaste.

Guided Meditation for Feeling More Beautiful

The more detached you are from your source, the more you obsess about your looks! The intrigue of the ego becomes deeply engrossed in our lives when we consistently attach our confidence level to our outer appearance. The ego wants you to be obsessed; the ego wants you to create a platform of outer expression that is based solely on the surface, not on your true inner beauty, or source. As I have said numerous times throughout the book, excessive attention to outer beauty tools and procedures that accommodate the needs of the ego will eventually leave you depleted to the point of denial or even depression. You must take action to force the ego to a standstill and eliminate the desire to use your outer looks to infuse yourself with a false set of beliefs. Self-love starts with the acceptance of who you truly are, and that begins by acknowledging the energy that you are made of.

Radical Recipe for Self-Love and True Beauty
Use Rose essential oil daily for seven days either in an essential oil burner or in a spray bottle with water and a few drops of witch hazel, and keep the essence in your home.

Remove all makeup and hair tools for seven days, and do not apply anything to yourself whatsoever.

Bring roses, or even better, buy a rose plant to have always in your home.

Use the Bach flower remedy Holly every day for seven days.

Meditation

Sit with your spine erect either in a chair or on a cushion.

Begin to breathe in and out through the nose, focusing on each breath. When your mind begins to stray, bring your attention immediately back to the breath.

When you begin to feel relaxed imagine your breath as a soothing light pink, or as the prettiest green you have ever seen!

Breathe in this light, and let it flow down into your heart centre or chakra.

Continue to breathe, and see only this light entering your body.

Be here and be still, and allow for the love you are made of to come forth.

When you are in a state of complete relaxation, repeat this affirmation to yourself:

I am beautiful just the way I am made.

I am strong and powerful.

I love myself and feel good about who I am.

I am love and I am living love everyday.

And so it is.

Use this practice whenever you are not feeling confident, have feelings of sadness or of not being good enough.

Guided Meditation for your Soul's Purpose

Deep beneath your worry and torment is your ever-flowing vibration of love waiting to come forth and guide you along life's most eminent journey. To get to the place that will lift you up day in and day out, you must first be willing to release all control to your ultimate self, which is your higher mind or higher self. Your higher self can be unlocked with the consistent and thoughtful practice of meditation. When you commit fully to a meditation practice, you are declaring to your higher self that you are now ready and willing to live the life you are meant to live. Allowing the flow of higher consciousness into your conscious mind may at first feel a little frightening to the ego. The key to effectively allowing the flow of your higher self involves resolving to relinquish any doubt you may have that your higher self or GOD truly exists within you. The absolute belief and conviction with your conscious mind that there is a higher power residing within you is all you need for the quest for enlightenment to begin.

Practice for Connecting to Your Higher Self
Sit comfortably with your spine erect either in a chair or on a comfortable cushion on the floor with your legs tucked in underneath you.

Recite this prayer:

Dear God,

I desire to know my true self.
I desire to live my soul's ultimate purpose.
I release unto you now all of my fear and my doubt.
I desire that you guide and direct me every day.
Please show me the direction in which I must turn now.
For I now know that as you lead the way, my life will become aligned with your desire for me.
And so it is.
Begin your session as follows and allow 20 minutes for the meditation.
Breathe in deeply.
Focus on the breath flowing in and out of the nose.
As you continue to focus on the breath, imagine the air that is flowing in and out as a white light.
Continue to see this white light flowing in and out of your nose.
As you breathe, keep the mind from wandering by focusing on your white light breath.
You will begin to relax enough to feel the energy of your higher self pulsating forward.
Remember to be patient and kind to yourself.

MIRROR MANTRAS

Mirror Mantras are an easy and effective way to affirmatively reprogram your thought patterns and brain frequency. Begin by looking in the mirror at yourself, and with compassion and love choose one of the mantras below to repeat to yourself daily. Practicing positive affirmations on a daily basis helps to assist you in activating your higher consciousness and reaffirms to your conscious mind that you are indeed a beautiful soul.

I believe in you!

You are beautiful!

And love lives and runs through you each and every moment!

My weight does not define me.

My true beauty pulsates from my heart

And uplifts everyone I encounter.

I am love,

I live love

And I am loving life today!

I am the new beauty!

You are beautiful and I love you!

Today I will live in the moment

And commit to feeling the beauty in me

And around me!

My face is sacred.

My body is sacred.

My soul is sacred.

My mind is sacred.

I am a sacred beauty.

I face my dear fear head-on and know that it comes from my ego,

Challenging me to embrace my own power and faith.

Today I know that all will be well

And everything is as it should be.

My beauty is full and strong!

Printed in the United States
By Bookmasters